HIGH TRIGLYCERIDE DIET HANDBOOK

WHAT TO EAT IF YOU HAVE TRIGLYCERIDE

CHASE ORCUTT

Table of Contents

CHAPTER ONE

High triglyceride diet

An unhealthy diet rich in triglyceride

To begin, what is triglyceride?

In your bloodstream, you'll find a fat called triglycerides.

When you eat, your body turns excess calories into triglycerides, which it stores in fat cells for later use as energy.

Levels of triglycerides

Even though triglycerides are an important source of energy for your body, a high level of triglycerides in the bloodstream increases your risk of heart disease. Triglyceride levels for adults are listed below in mg/dL (milligrams per deciliter).

Triglyceride levels over 150 mg/dL are considered elevated in approximately 25.9% of adults in the United States.

Alcohol consumption and a high-calorie diet, combined with obesity or poorly controlled diabetes, can raise triglyceride levels in the blood.

Ways to reduce triglyceride levels.

A variety of dietary and lifestyle modifications can help lower your triglyceride levels.

Aim for a weight that is appropriate for your height and activity level.

Overeating causes your body to produce triglycerides, which it then stores as fat in your cells.

If you want to lower your blood triglyceride levels, you should try to maintain a healthy weight.

A recent study found that even a small amount of weight loss can have a significant impact on triglyceride levels.

Triglyceride levels in the blood can be permanently lowered by losing at least 5% of your body weight.

Consume sugar in moderation.

Many people's diets include a significant amount of added sugar.

A study found that the average American consumed 308 calories of added sugar daily, despite the American Heart Association's recommendation of no more than 100–150 calories per day.

Sweets, soft drinks, and fruit juice all contain added sugar.

Having too much sugar in your diet can lead to an increase in blood triglyceride levels and other risk factors for heart disease.

A 2020 study of 6,730 people found that those who regularly drank sugar-sweetened beverages had triglyceride levels that were more than twice as likely to be high as those who did not.

Children who consume a lot of added sugar are more likely to develop high blood triglyceride levels.

Fortunately, several studies have shown that a reduction in triglyceride levels in the blood can be achieved by following a low carb diet.

Some people's triglycerides can be reduced with as little as a switch to water from sugar-sweetened beverages.

Sugary drinks and sweets can raise your blood triglyceride levels if you consume too much of them.

Reduce your carbohydrate intake.

As with added sugar, extra calories from carbs in your diet are converted into triglycerides and stored in fat cells, just like the extra sugar.

For those who want to lower their triglyceride levels, low-carb diets have been shown to do so.

At six, twelve, and twenty-four months, a meta-analysis of 12 randomized controlled trials found that people on low-carb diets typically saw their triglyceride levels drop. Triglyceride levels decreased the most six months after beginning a low-calorie diet in these studies.

Low-fat and low-carb diets were compared in a 2020 study. Researchers discovered that those on a low-carb diet saw greater reductions in triglyceride levels than those on a low-fat diet 6–12 months after starting their respective diets.

Chapter two

In the short term, a low-carb diet can reduce blood triglyceride levels significantly, compared to a low-fat diet.

Consume a greater quantity of fiber.

Fruits, vegetables, and whole grains all contain dietary fiber in naturally occurring forms, making them excellent sources for a healthy diet. Nuts, seeds, cereals, and legumes are also rich sources of the nutrient.

A diet high in fiber can help lower your triglyceride levels by slowing the absorption of fat and sugar in the small intestine.

A study of 117 overweight or obese adults found that those who ate more dietary fiber had lower triglyceride levels.

Consuming a high-fiber cereal with an oily breakfast reduced the amount of fat in the blood by 50% in adolescents, according to another small study.

Your blood triglyceride levels may be reduced by increasing the amount of fiber in your diet from fruits, vegetables, and whole grains.

Regularly work out.

Triglycerides can be reduced by combining aerobic exercise with weight loss, according to research.

This recommendation is from the American Heart Association, which states that adults should engage in at least 30 minutes of aerobic exercise at least five days per week.

The long-term effects of exercise on triglyceride levels are most apparent. A study in people with heart disease found that exercising 45 minutes a day, five days a week reduced blood triglycerides by a significant amount.

Triglyceride levels can be reduced by any form of exercise. Research has shown that exercising at a higher intensity for a shorter period of time is more effective than exercising at a moderate intensity for a longer period of time.

Regular high-intensity aerobic exercise may improve HDL (good) cholesterol levels and lower blood triglyceride levels if done on a regular basis.

Avoid trans fats at all costs

To extend the shelf life of processed foods, artificial trans fats are used.

Partially hydrogenated oils, which are commonly used in

commercially fried foods and baked goods, contain trans fats. Some animal products also contain small amounts of them. Trans fats have been banned in the United States in recent years.

Trans fats have been linked to a variety of health issues, including elevated levels of LDL (bad) cholesterol and heart disease, due to their pro-inflammatory properties.

According to a meta-analysis of 16 studies, swapping trans fats for polyunsaturated fats can lower blood triglyceride levels (26).

Consuming large amounts of trans fats can raise both blood triglyceride levels and the risk of heart disease. Limiting your intake of highly processed and fried foods can help reduce your trans fat intake.

twice a week eat fatty fish

The health benefits of fatty fish, including its ability to lower blood triglycerides, are well-known.

Omega-3 fatty acids, a type of polyunsaturated fatty acid that is considered essential, are the primary reason why this fish is so beneficial..

Eating two servings of fatty fish a week is recommended by both the Dietary Guidelines for Americans and the American Heart Association.

Moreover, a study found that eating salmon twice a week significantly reduced blood triglyceride concentration.

Some of the best sources of omega-3 fatty acids include salmon, sardines, tuna, and mackerel.

Omega-3 fatty acids can be found in fatty fish such as tuna and salmon. Reduce triglyceride levels and heart disease risk by eating two servings per week.

Unsaturated fats should be consumed in greater amounts.

The replacement of carbs with monounsaturated and polyunsaturated fats has been shown to lower blood triglyceride levels.

Olive oil, nuts, and avocados, for example, are rich in monounsaturated fats. Vegetable oils and fatty fish, as well as nuts and seeds like walnuts, flaxseeds, and chia seeds, all contain polyunsaturated fats.

Olive oil consumption does lower triglyceride levels, but at a lower rate than other plant oils, according to a 2019 review of 27 studies.

An older study examined the 24-hour diets of 452 adults from an Alaskan Indigenous population.

According to the study, those who consumed more saturated fat were more likely to have an increased risk for high triglyceride levels in their blood.

Instead of trans fats or highly processed vegetable oils, try substituting heart-healthy olive oil for the triglyceride-lowering benefits of unsaturated fats.

Chapter three

It is possible to lower blood triglyceride levels by consuming monounsaturated and polyunsaturated fats instead of other fats.

Establish a consistent meal schedule.

In addition, insulin resistance can contribute to elevated blood triglycerides.

The cells in your pancreas receive a signal after a meal that tells them to release insulin into your bloodstream. Your cells use sugar as a source of energy, and insulin is responsible for transporting it to them.

Too much insulin in the bloodstream can cause insulin resistance, which makes it difficult for the body to use insulin efficiently.. Sugar and triglyceride levels in the blood may rise as a result of this.

Establishing a regular eating schedule can mitigate the effects of insulin resistance and high triglyceride levels, which is good news. It's been discovered, for example, that skipping breakfast can reduce one's insulin sensitivity in the body.

According to a statement from the American Heart Association, eating irregularly lowers one's chances of achieving healthy cardiometabolic levels. They advocated eating on a regular schedule and planning your meals ahead of time.

In terms of meal frequency, however, the evidence is a little less clear.

A 2013 study found that eating three meals a day instead of six meals a day significantly reduced triglycerides.

Several other studies, on the other hand, suggest that altering the frequency of meals has little impact on triglyceride levels.

Maintaining a regular meal schedule can improve insulin sensitivity and lower blood triglyceride levels, no matter how many meals you eat each day.

A regular meal schedule has been shown to reduce the risk of heart disease and insulin resistance, despite a lack of conclusive research on the subject.

Do not overindulge in alcoholic beverages.

Many alcoholic beverages are loaded with sugar, carbohydrates, and calories, making them an unhealthy choice. Triglycerides can be stored in fat cells if these calories remain unutilized.

Triglycerides are transported into your system via very large very low density lipoproteins (VLDLs), which are increased in the liver by alcohol.

Moderate alcohol consumption has been shown to increase blood triglycerides by up to 53%, even if your triglyceride levels are already normal.

The consumption of light to moderate amounts of alcohol has been linked with a lower risk for heart disease, while binge drinking has been linked to an increased risk.

Limiting alcohol consumption may help lower triglyceride levels in the blood, according to some research.

Add soy protein to your daily diet

Isoflavones, a type of plant compound that has numerous health benefits, are found in soy. Soy protein has been shown to lower blood triglyceride levels, despite its well-known role in lowering LDL (bad) cholesterol.

A meta-analysis of 46 studies found that postmenopausal women who regularly consumed soy protein had significantly lower triglyceride levels.

Soybeans (edamame), tofu, tempeh, and soy milk all contain soy protein.

Compounds in soy have been linked to numerous health benefits. Soy protein may help lower blood triglycerides by replacing animal protein.

Eat more nuts from the tree.

The fiber, omega-3 fatty acids, and unsaturated fats in tree nuts help lower triglycerides in the blood.

Each daily serving of tree nuts was found to lower triglyceride levels by an average of 2.2 mg/dL (0.02 mmol/l) in one analysis.

Tree nut consumption was linked to a small reduction in triglycerides in another review of 49 studies.

Nuts found in trees include:

* almonds

* pecans

* walnuts

* cashews

* pistachios

* Brazil nut butter

* macadamia nut butters

Nuts, on the other hand, are a good source of calories. Moderation is key when it comes to eating almonds, as a serving of 23 almonds has 164 calories.

Nut consumption of 3–7 servings per week has been found to have the greatest health benefits in most studies.

Fibre, omega-3 fatty acids, and unsaturated fats are just a few of the heart-healthy nutrients found in nuts. Eating 3–7 servings of tree nuts per week may help lower blood triglycerides, according to research.

Ask your doctor if there are any natural supplements that could benefit you.

A number of natural supplements may have the ability to reduce blood triglyceride levels, according to research. Consult with your doctor before taking any supplements, as they may interact with other medications.

The Food and Drug Administration (FDA) does not regulate supplements in the same manner as it regulates pharmaceuticals, and supplement quality can vary greatly.

The following are some of the most commonly studied supplements:

• Fish oil Many studies have shown that omega-3 fatty acids found in fish oil can help lower triglycerides and other risk factors for cardiovascular disease.

• Fenugreek. Fenugreek seeds have long been used to increase milk production, but recent studies have shown that they can also help lower blood triglycerides.

Vitamin D is an important source of this vitamin. Supplementing with vitamin D has been shown to help lower triglyceride levels in the body as a whole.

• Curcumin. A review of seven studies found that curcumin supplementation could reduce triglyceride and LDL (bad) cholesterol levels.

Fish oil, fenugreek, garlic extract, guggul, and curcumin

have all been studied for their ability to lower triglyceride levels.

The nitty-gritty

Triglyceride levels can be significantly influenced by dietary and lifestyle choices.

Trans fats should be replaced with healthy, unsaturated fats, carbohydrates and added sugars should be reduced, and regular exercise should be incorporated into your daily routine.

You can lower your triglycerides and improve your health in general by making a few simple lifestyle changes.

There's no need to drastically alter your eating habits or way of life all at once. For long-term, sustainable changes that are easier to maintain, experiment with some of the tips listed above and gradually incorporate other strategies into your daily routine.

THE END